THE SELF-CARE SURVIVAL GUIDE FOR EMPLOYEES

Simple tips to help you avoid burnout and show up for life (and work) radically happier and healthier

Misty Hudek Giordano

Beginning Gratitude

This book is dedicated to you, for your willingness and excitement to choose a different path for yourself and to inspire those around you, just by doing so.

You inspire me.

Table of Contents

Intention 1

Chapter 1 - Authentic Movement 8

Chapter 2 - Food as Fuel 20

Chapter 3 - Self-Care as Healthcare 29

Chapter 4 - Rest as Medicine 50

Chapter 5 - Preparation for Sanity 68

Chapter 6 - Zen Your Space for Calm Clarity 75

Chapter 7 - BONUS! Self-Care in a Pinch 88

Help! I'm Overwhelmed with Options!! 94

Resources the Author Recommends 95

Ending Gratitude 98

Dedication 100

Intention

Once upon a time, I worked in an office setting - much like the one you might find yourself in right now. During my 10 years working in that particular office, I was faced with so many health challenges. Just like a lot of other work environments, there was no shortage of stress, busyness and a general lack of proactive self-care on my end. I grew up the daughter of a woman who worked 2-3 jobs to support her family and literally ran her health into the gutter. Family patterns.

The truth is, there's nothing unusual about that story. Most of us operate our lives in survival mode day in and day out. We're juggling life, careers, relationships, kids, other jobs, ailing parents, money issues and a slew of other concerns. Very often, we find our own self-care on the backburner - blazing bright, but just waiting for that inevitable block to remove itself - time. Having and/or finding the time to get to it.

After I left that office job to go off on my own into the professional wellness field, I really started to see the merging of the two worlds together. I had been building and growing my own business in tandem with that office job for about 4 years, and in those 4 years I was exposed to a whole new world of possibilities in holistic medicine and lifestyle modifications. Self-care, herbs, plants, food as fuel; I started absorbing and learning as much as I could. I couldn't get enough - anytime I found something fascinating, down the rabbit hole I went to learn as much as I could. I started thinking about how much I didn't know before and how it could've made such a difference when it came to my health. So many of these things I was learning could have been implemented during my office time to counteract different physical and emotional challenges I was going through, both from the job itself and from other life factors. Let's face it - life is rarely ever completely smooth-sailing. There's no shortage of stress in day to day life, and all that takes its toll on the body - maybe not right away, but over time.

I started realizing that we talk and teach so much about things to do when you're at home, on the weekends, on our own time - things like exercising, eating good food, taking time to disconnect, family time, etc. and while that's amazing, most people I know spend the majority of their lives at work. Work can be in an office setting, in the field, in a remote setting, a coworking space, working from home, in a hospital, in a church, at a non-profit or anything else. I saw a giant disconnect between the "home" self-care and the self-care we were able to partake in for ourselves during work hours.

Originally when I was inspired to write this book, I thought I would be writing it for the employer and human resource departments of companies – afterall, changing the wellness in the workplace initiatives in companies would be a huge benefit. After seeing how simple and easy some of these things could be, how could they go back to doing things a different way? However, the truth is, workplace wellness is still emerging as a new idea - most companies still think of it as an idea that's slowly making the rounds, or something that is in its infancy. Most workplace wellness programs really hit exercising hard, giving precedence to apps and guidance on things to do to move the body. Some incorporate food choices. These are all great things, and I'm by no means trying to take anything away from what has been created or what you currently have access to. However, there's so much more available to you.

My intention for this book now is to ensure it gets it into the hands of all employees, everywhere. **What I've noticed with myself and with those I've had the pleasure to work with is that we tend to look to others to fix us, help us, save us, make life better in some way.** We do this most often in the work environment because we feel a bit like a puppet that doesn't get much say in how things go and how the ship is sailed. We're just along for the ride and dancing to the beat of our employer's drum. What if I told you that this isn't actually completely true though?

A truly pivotal awareness in my life was realizing that we are the creator of our lives. Workplace wellness and culture all play a really integral role, for sure, but at the end of the day there is actually so much we could be doing for ourselves on all levels - physically, emotionally, spiritually, etc. regardless where we physically find ourselves.

Let's use the metaphor of a car as it pertains to yourself, your life and your health. You know that for a car to run it needs to be cared for and fueled up. Without these things, the car will break down, stall, and burn out. Our bodies on every layer are the same. If we're constantly giving without replenishing, it won't be long before we completely burn out. Burnout can take many forms, including physical and/or emotional burnout and can often lead to disease.

My invitation to you is to first become aware of this cycle in your own life and then take some proactive steps to lessen the effects of your circumstances - where in your life are you over-giving without replenishing? Are you feeling burnt out, and if so, to what extent?

The core intention of this book is to give you ideas of things you CAN do - often times right now - that can help you really connect with your body and give it what it's asking you for and being able to give those things to yourself in a way that won't get you in trouble with your employer. This book is by no means exhaustive of all the options available to you - that would be impossible. In fact, some of the greatest self-care techniques I've practiced for myself have come by way of taking an idea that was presented to me and expanding upon it to make it authentic to me and what I need - like creating your own self-care adventure. It needs to be mentioned that all of these options may not be feasible or doable in your current employment situation, so make sure you're aware of what is acceptable by management and appropriate in your situation.

The idea of the practices mentioned in this book are things that are either free or lower in cost - I'm not a huge fan of spending tons of money on self-care. It's great and all, but it usually isn't sustainable in the long haul. We're looking for consistency - quick and easy things you can do daily or almost every day, regardless of the resources at your disposal.

I invite you to absorb from the book what you will, integrate some things into your life slowly - one by one. Do one until you know it works for you, until you can actually see and feel the benefits, until it becomes a habit and then add another one. I'm not an advocate of fire-hosing yourself with this whole new, lofty, badass self-care routine. Good intentions, sure, but what I'm inviting you to incorporate into your life is ease and consistency. My definition of self-care is any practice that helps elevate you from wherever you are now to a greater sense of calm, meaning something that is sustainable and not yet another item on your mile-long to-do list. When things become a "have to do," they can become stressful and can trigger anxiety. That's the opposite of what I'm inviting you to. So be aware of yourself and your body, listen to your intuition, go with what your body needs regardless of whether it looks like something in this book or not. Most likely, whatever your new self-care habits end up looking like, they might be far different from that of your coworkers, friends, family and mine. Try to treat self-care as a bit of a self-discovery adventure. Allow this book to be a springboard to do a little digging on your end into the things that really interest you - learn more about them, find people who specialize in that particular modality, access the plethora of resources available to you - you may just find your new passion in your self-care routine.

One last thing - don't be surprised if you start inspiring other people around you just by taking your self-care seriously in your own life and workplace. The best way to be a living, breathing example to other people - our coworkers, our kids, our family, our friends, everyone - is to dive so deep into our own self-love and health, cultivate our authenticity and really turn inward to create stillness and peace in any situation that your radiant energy can't help but ripple out to the people around you. *Leading by example, now that's inspiring.*

With so much love and gratitude,

Misty

PS – It also needs to be mentioned that I'm not a medical professional of any kind and the information and resources contained in this book are not intended to diagnose, treat, prevent or cure any physical or emotional ailment or provide any kind of medical advice. If you have a medical concern or question, you should consult with your health care provider or seek other professional medical treatment.

Chapter 1 - Authentic Movement

We're going to dive right in with the one thing a lot of workplace wellness programs usually include; movement and exercise. Yes, I know - the word might bring up memories of that time your office did "the biggest loser" challenge. Or the time you signed up for that 5k you thought you'd crush but it ended up crushing you instead - or worse, you got scared because you didn't train so you bailed on the race even after you paid the money, just to save yourself the embarrassment. I may have personal experience in all of those. Whatever emotions the words "movement" and "exercise" conjure up for you, I would love for you to just let those go for now in lieu of openness to new possibilities.

We tend to look at exercising in a specific light - it reminds us of things such as yoga, running, weight lifting, etc. All great things, if that's what you're into. The idea of this chapter though is to introduce you to some, perhaps, unconventional means of moving your body within the work environment and beyond. Some of these ideas might only work in great weather, so if you live in a climate that is extremely cold or extremely hot, you'll have to adjust accordingly and maybe find a new, better option for those months of the year. Again, allow these ideas to be a springboard to zoom out and widen your awareness of different possibilities beyond the norm. Get creative!

A prelude to these chapters - the way I'll set these up for you is to introduce the practice or idea, give you a small idea on why it works and some tips on how to do it. At the end of each chapter will be a worksheet where you can write down (or even just use them as prompts to ponder on) notes, takeaways, what stood out to you, what you really got jazzed about incorporating into your life, etc. Some chapters will also include an interview from someone I consider an expert in that particular field - I have so many people I consider health ninjas. This is just a small sampling, but they have some amazing perspectives to share!

For this chapter, the question you might be asking yourself is, "How can I get movement in my day when I'm stuck in an office for 8 or more hours?"

Some ideas:

Stretching

Why?

Stretching can increase your flexibility and range of motion, sure, but it can also increase the blood flow to your muscles, help prevent back pain (like from sitting for long periods of time) and it's really great for stress relief and to calm your mind.

<u>How?</u>

While I'd imagine getting into a downward dog position or child's pose might warrant some curious stares from management or neighboring cubicles, you can absolutely do a few stretches either in your chair or by standing up. Everything always starts with intention, so one thing I would invite you to do before you decide how to stretch is to close your eyes for a minute and feel into your body - where are you feeling tight? Where are you holding stress? We tend to spend a lot of time hunched over a phone or a computer, so a counter stretch could be opening your arms and reaching a little backwards to really open up your chest and expand instead of contract. If your lower back is tight, maybe stand up and take a forward bend to stretch out your back and legs. Be aware of your own body, stretching should feel good and not be painful. Allow your body to tell you what it needs and don't push it beyond its limits.

Utilize your lunch break in a new way

<u>Why?</u>

Time and time again what a lot of people tend to do is take their lunch breaks in the office lunchroom, at their desks or in their cars, which equals more sitting. While moving your body has so many benefits, one that I love to reap while taking a mid-day movement break is the decrease in stress it provides while lifting your mood.

How?

What if you spent your lunch hour incorporating some movement before you ate lunch? Depending on where you work and how much time you have, you may have a local gym or yoga studio that's close, maybe your workplace even has a gym, or you live close to your house. Maybe see if there's a way you can make a trip there on your lunch break and get some movement in. If that isn't an option, maybe finding a quiet and/or open space to do some stretching, yoga postures, taking a walk or some other variation of using your lunch hour to include some movement might be more your speed. If your workplace has stairs nearby or in the building, taking a few rounds up and down could be another idea.

Dancing

Why?

Because duh, who doesn't dance at work? Seriously though, this one might not be feasible, but it deserves an honorable mention for those who might be able to sneak it in somehow. Moving your body, as I've mentioned before, can help reduce stress and anxiety, but dancing in particular can actually move energy out of the body. What does that mean? Ever have one of those days where you're just kind of meh, or even worse not having a super stellar day and you just need to shake it off? Dancing can help with that. Dancing can literally help move all that gunky energy out of the body to make way for more positive energy to come in.

<u>How?</u>

Put on a really great song and dance around in whichever way the spirit moves you (and doesn't land you in the HR office). Fast, slow, ecstatic, flowy, whatever works for you. I've been known to get in my truck and take a drive to really let loose, I may or may not have had many solo dance parties in the (private) bathroom in my old company as well. Remember, I'm not advocating for anything, I'm just simply giving you some ideas and telling stories of what I've done in my day =)

Walking Meetings

<u>Why?</u>

I love this idea and I so wish more places got on board with this. If you're in a management position and you're able to institute this, or suggest it to management, it could mean a whole different level of helping your crew get out of the office, get some fresh air and improve their mental clarity (amongst other things I've already mentioned). You may also find everyone coming up with more creative solutions to problems while they're outside!

<u>How?</u>

In lieu of your normal conference room meeting, move it outside, weather permitting! Walk and talk, sit outside and talk, make your own variation of this while being cognizant of those who may have physical limitations. There are options to play with here.

Walking Lunch

<u>Why?</u>

Walking can energize you, it gets you outside into the natural sunlight and gets your body moving in a way that isn't exhausting and won't leave you too sweaty. It can also allow you to really disconnect from the work environment and de-stress.

<u>How?</u>

Go outside. Walk. This one is pretty self-explanatory!

<u>Expert Interview</u>

Nicole Wolfe, Head of Corporate Programs at ClassPass

<u>About:</u>

Founded in 2013, ClassPass is the world's most flexible network of fitness and wellness experiences. Members gain instant access to over 22,000 pre-vetted exercise studios, which offer diverse fitness options including yoga, cycling, Pilates, strength training, boxing and more. In addition to workouts, members can instantly book inspiring wellness experiences and beauty-treatments that go beyond fitness, such as massages, acupuncture, spa treatments, hydrotherapy, and post-workout blowouts. Recognized as one of Forbes' Next Billion Dollar Startups, ClassPass simplifies the discovery process, using machine learning to provide catered recommendations to each member based on their goals and preferences. Just search for a class or experience, reserve your spot, and go. More information can be found at corporate.classpass.com

<u>Interview:</u>

What ramifications for a lack of self-care do you see most often in workplace settings?

A CareerBuilder survey found that 1/3 employees feel high stress levels at work. As a result, employees are experiencing symptoms including anxiety, weight gain, poor sleep, depression and weakened immune systems, leading to more burnout and sick days. Employees should be given tools to help manage their health and wellness, and need to feel that employers prioritize their wellbeing.

What method of self-care do you personally feel is most important and/or effective for the general population, especially as it pertains to something they can do in the workplace setting?

At ClassPass, we've developed a corporate wellness program that provides discounted and subsidized memberships for employees. Those who opt into the program are offered access to more than 22,000 boutique studios and gyms worldwide. Our social features encourage employees to go to class together and increase camaraderie, motivation and culture. The reason ClassPass works is because employees are given the tools to find the classes and experiences that work around their schedules and goals. Employees can opt for morning yoga classes to find their Zen before the start of the day, head to a lunchtime HIIT class with colleagues, or work off any workday frustrations in an 8pm boxing class.

In your ideal world, what would workplace wellness look like in every company?

Wellness is not a one-size-fits-all approach. Understanding the unique needs of employees is critical to any wellness program, which is why there needs to be variety and flexibility.This includes things like leadership participation, supporting employees' grassroots efforts and providing solutions for employees across the spectrum (demographics, location, career path, etc.).

Chapter 1 - Ponderments

Notes, ah-ha's, braindumps, moments of clarity, interesting ideas:

What is an easy way to incorporate more movement into your work day?

Is there anything you can foresee that might get in the way of this? What can you do to avoid that potential roadblock?

Chapter 2 - Food as Fuel

Darn the office with their deliciously irresistible sugary treats that call to you from the office lunchroom. Coooooommmmmeeee toooo meeeeee Sarah! It's like a scene from a bad zombie movie and something I fell victim to every dang time! I know I'm not alone there and I know it's something that's a constant struggle. How do you keep on top of your food game when the whole office is noshing on donuts, pastries, catered in meals laden with fried foods, fast food and everything in between?!

The bad news is, it's not easy. I'm not one to beat around the bush, especially not with you. If you're like me, you have a serious problem saying no to really yummy things when they're right in your face. The health coach in me is going to tell you not to cut yourself off completely, but just make mindful choices of what is REALLY going to taste amazing. I think we can all relate to that thing that looked really amazing, it smelled really amazing, but the taste was anything but amazing, but you didn't want to be wasteful so you ate it anyway, and then you were mad because you ate such an unhealthy thing that wasn't even good and now you feel like crap when it allllllllll could've been avoided by just throwing it out! Am I right?!

Either way, you might be asking yourself, "How can I eat better while being surrounded by junk food and temptation?" Here are some ideas to help you stay on top of fueling your body with good, clean food even without disturbing the peace with the rest of the office.

Meal Prep

<u>Why?</u>

Meal prepping is a huge time saver. It was an idea that I bucked for so long, and then once I started, I couldn't figure out how I made anything else work before. The idea of meal prepping is making your lunch and/or dinner for a few days ahead of time so it's ready to go with you to work rather than spending time every day making the day's meals.

<u>How?</u>

Usually people take one day, most often a weekend day, to spend a few hours in the kitchen prepping their lunches and/or dinners for the week. Yes, this takes some weekend time away, BUT you're gaining lots of weekday time back. Think about how awesome it would feel not to have to worry about what you're going to have for lunch or dinner tomorrow! If you need some ideas, hop on Pinterest and type in something like "meal prep recipes" in the search. Some people choose one thing to eat the entire week, some people make a variety of things. Some people do easy salads, some people do crockpot meals, while some make simple sandwiches. This can be as unique as you are, as simple or as extravagant as you'd like. No right or wrong here, it's just what works for you. Depending on what you're making and for how many days, sometimes packing half of it away in the freezer and then thawing it out the day before is a great idea to preserve the freshness, because while meal prepping is amazing, the food that's been sitting in the fridge for 4 or 5 days might get a little.... ewww.

Meal Prep/Delivery Service

Why?

Because sometimes the idea of meal prepping is too much for people to handle, or they don't even like cooking. I enlist the help of a weekly meal service to make sure I always have fresh, prepared food available no matter what my schedule might throw at me.

How?

Get to Google and search out some companies that can cater to your dietary needs (paleo, vegetarian, keto, gluten free, vegan, etc.), food selection preferences (like organic vs. conventional) and whether or not they deliver to your area or offer a pickup hub. While some services might have a sticker shock value associated with them, I invite you to consider that you're reinvesting the money you would've been spending in the grocery store on food for the week into a service that's cooking for you, like a personal chef of sorts. This doesn't take into account the cost of your time either; time is a precious resource we can never put a dollar value on. To each their own here!

Keep a Healthier Sweet Treat at the Ready

Why?

Because who wants to feel left out when the whole office is mowing down donuts and you're sitting there salivating watching it all happen?! That's no fun for anyone.

How?

Find something that is decadent and deliciously healthy for those days when the sugar cravings are just too much to handle. Dark chocolate, seasoned almonds, trail mix with some chocolate pieces in it; whatever feels like a treat to you, but won't send you spiraling into a brain fog and spending the rest of the day in regret. Here's a hint - if you have a self-control problem with sweets (perhaps like, oh I don't know, me) and you fear that if you buy it, you're going to eat it all the same day - have a coworker hide it somewhere for you and when the donuts arrive, ask them to magically unhide the thing without you knowing where they were hidden so they can be safely put back for the next time. Just in case though, if you take this route, you may want to let 2 coworkers in on the secret hiding place, just in case one happens to be off that day! Better safe than sorry, these instances are no laughing matter.

Communal Lunch

Why?

In some countries, there's this really cool practice they do in their communities where each family cooks for the whole community once per month. That might sound like a huge undertaking, but when you factor in that the other 27-30 days of the month, you're having your meal made for you, that doesn't sound half bad! So, I got to thinking, how cool would something like this be in an office setting?

How?

Get a group of coworkers together and see if you can divide up the work week lunches. If there are 5 of you, you each take a day and make a healthy lunch for your group and you rotate. You provide for one day, they provide the other days. If there's more than 5, you can create this as you wish. For example, if there's 10 people who want to commit to this, maybe you provide lunch once every two weeks, or maybe you partner up and split the cost and/or work (i.e. if you're bringing tacos, maybe you make the filling and the other brings the tortillas and toppings). Granted, let's be honest, you need to make sure whomever is included in this is reliable to come through on their day with their duties. The idea is to share the load, not be one of the only ones contributing, so choose your people wisely. This is something that can be accommodating for different dietary needs too - like in the example above, if you have a vegetarian in the group, maybe make extra veggies for them to fill their tacos with. If you have someone who is gluten free, perhaps you can split the tortilla options between corn and flour.

Chapter 2 - Ponderments

Notes, ah-ha's, braindumps, moments of clarity, interesting ideas:

What is an easy way to help support feeding your body with good fuel sources?

Is there anything you can foresee that might get in the way of this? What can you do to avoid that potential roadblock?

____

____

____

____

____

____

____

____

____

____

____

____

____

____

____

____

Chapter 3 - Self-Care as Healthcare

It would be an abomination if we didn't spend a big chunk of this book talking about specific practices that could help you up your self-care game, both at home and in the office. Obviously, the practices thus far are great ideas, but you might be wondering how you can best disengage from what's happening at work and settle your mind and your body during the day and at the end of your day. Here are some ideas that will help with just that!

Use these ideas to start, end or take a break during your day and remember - expand on these ideas and be open to seeking out other options that might be waiting for you!

Self-Massage

Why?

Along with stretching, massaging sore and tight muscles can help loosen and relieve tension. If you're at home, you can make this into a bit of a more luxurious self-massage by using a lotion with clean ingredients or something simple like coconut oil.

How?

Notice where you're holding some tightness and tension - is it your neck? Your shoulders? Your low back? Your hips? Wherever you're feeling it, gently massage those areas for a bit to help loosen the muscles and assist with blood flow. This can be done in your office, in your chair, car, the bathroom, anywhere that suits you. To kick it up a notch, utilize an essential oil that can help relieve and soothe muscle tension (like lavender or peppermint, for example).

Tech Disconnect

Why?

This is one of my absolute favorite (and easiest, but hardest!) methods of self-care. A technology disconnect is quite literally moving away from anything that qualifies as technology for a prolonged period of time - be it minutes, hours or even days in some cases with some devices. All day long our lives are ruled by technology; from computers to smart phones to smart watches to TV's to video games to microwaves. It's my theory that technology is quite literally turning us into robots and disconnecting us from ourselves, each other, the Earth; all of it. While tech is here to stay, it doesn't need to rule our lives.

How?

Step awaaaaay from the screens. Literally. Take a break and leave anything tech inside (and locked up if that needs to be the case). Go outside, leave your phone, your smart watch, anything that makes noise or vibrates or has a screen - leave it somewhere you aren't going to be. All the electromagnetic waves and screen time isn't doing us, our bodies or our internal systems (our nervous system especially!) a kindness. I love doing social media detoxes. Want to see how much time you actually have in any given day? Stay off social media for a week and see what happens to your mood and how much free time you magically have in your life!

Earthing

Why?

Ok this one might be a little out there for some of you, but hear me out - you're going to love it! The good people over at www.barefoothealing.com.au explained Earthing so well. "Years of extensive research has shown that connecting to the Earth's natural energy, by walking barefoot on grass, sand, dirt or rock can diminish chronic pain, fatigue and other ailments that plague so many people today. This connection is referred to as Earthing or Grounding. To put it briefly, when your bare feet or skin comes in contact with the Earth, free electrons are taken up into the body. These electrons could be referred to as nature's biggest antioxidants and help neutralize damaging excess free radicals that can lead to inflammation and disease in the body. The Earth is a conductor for free electrons and so are all living things on the planet, including us. The body is composed mostly of water and minerals, which in combination are excellent conductors of electrons from the Earth, provided there is direct skin contact or some other conductive channel for them to flow through. The Earth's energy upgrades one's physiology by allowing the body to cope and repair thereby promoting wellbeing, vitality and better sleep. It also harmonizes and stabilizes the body's basic biological rhythms, knocks down (and even knocks out) chronic inflammation and reduces and eliminates associated pain, making it the most natural and powerful anti-inflammatory and anti-aging remedy around!"

<u>How?</u>

If there's grass nearby, go outside and take your shoes off. It doesn't have to be a huge, lush acre of grass - any grass will do (preferably grass that isn't treated with any kind of pesticides though, you don't want to walk on that stuff and have it get into your body through the pores on your feet!). If grass isn't near, find a tree and place your hands on the tree. If you don't have grass or a tree, but you have a natural body of water or sand, put your feet and/or hands in the sand or water. Regardless what conductor I'm using, what I love doing is leaving everything technological somewhere else (see above for the tech disconnect methods) and going outside all by myself, somewhere peaceful where you won't be bothered - or aren't likely to be bothered. With my bare hands/feet touching the Earth in some capacity, I love using my breath in conjunction with this practice - as you inhale, imagine you're breathing in all the positive emotions you want to feel (peace, joy, happiness, contentment, whatever it is - breathe in those emotions into your body and let it fill you). As you exhale, imagine sending any unwanted emotions or pain into the Earth. Keep doing this for as long as time will allow. The more time you can spend in nature, the better you'll feel!

Nature time

Why?

Nature is good for the soul. Fresh air is amazing for your body and your systems, getting out into the natural elements can be so incredible for the body (reread the benefits of the Earthing section). When we're cooped up in an office all day breathing in the same recirculated air, being blasted with the air conditioning or heat, our bodies are literally craving fresh air, being out in the sunlight and just being outdoors.

<u>How?</u>

Refer to the section on movement - specifically about taking walks on your lunch break. Even if you don't want to take a walk or can't for whatever reason, just going outside to have lunch or take a break in the grass or amongst the trees can do wonders for your body and your mood alike. Another idea is to open up your windows (if you can) in your office, car, home, etc. to let out the stagnant air and allow fresh air to filter in. If you have windows that open in your office though, be sure to anchor down any papers before the wind blows them all over your office like in the movies :).

Meditation

<u>Why?</u>

Did you think you were going to read a self-care book and meditation would NOT be mentioned? Come on now! Here's the truth though - you don't have to contort your body into a pretzel, close your eyes and chant "Om" to meditate. That's for sure one way to do it, and if that floats your boat then that's just fabulous! If it isn't though, just know that sitting quietly by yourself with your eyes closed, if only for 5 minutes, to focus on clearing your mind of all the thoughts, emotions and anxieties you might be feeling is a great way to infuse some meditation into your day.

<u>How?</u>

There's no right or wrong way to do this, but some ideas might be finding a guided meditation you can listen to on a break. Find a good spot to go – could be your office, lunchroom, car, wherever - and pop some earbuds in. YouTube is full of really great short, free guided meditations if you'd like to go that route. If earbuds and a guided meditation are totally out of the question for whatever reason, you can absolutely just sit quietly with your eyes closed or open and try to clear your mind. When I was first starting out, what I would focus on was a movie screen just before the previews would come on, when it was totally blank. For every thought that would come into my head and thus onto the movie screen, I'd imagine big hands pushing it to the sides of the screen while I focused on the blank screen. You can use this in tandem with the next section on breathing.

Breathing

<u>Why?</u>

The practice of mindful breathing has so many benefits, but two of the ones I want to highlight here are improving brain function and boosting energy levels. I love this practice because you don't need to go anywhere to do this, you can do this at any time, right at your desk or anywhere else.

<u>How?</u>

There are many variations, but I love keeping things simple and building upon it from there. Take a 5 count on each inhale and exhale - breathe in for 5 counts, filling up your belly, your midsection and your lungs, hold it in for 5 seconds and then exhale for 5 seconds letting as much air out as you can. I like having my eyes closed for this, it helps me stay in the moment and in my breath. If you want to go longer, you can up it to 6 counts, then 7, maybe 10. Go with what feels good to you and pay attention to what happens to your body once you get to a certain repetition. Maybe on breath 5 your shoulders all of a sudden soften. Perhaps at breath 3 your heart begins to slow down. Maybe on breath 8 your chest starts to expand even more. Keep leaning into what feels good to you and do these as often as you need.

Natural remedies at work

<u>Why?</u>

Our bodies are constantly under attack each and every day from invaders of all shapes and sizes. If we think about our bodies and all the systems we house, it's amazing to think about all the things it does for us without us even realizing it. Your immune system is protecting you from germs and viruses that you're exposed to from other people, public places, things you're touching, etc. Your digestive system is breaking down your food so your body can absorb and use all the good nutrients to build up your other systems. Your respiratory system is breathing for you without you having to tell it to (I mean really, how cool is that?). When one of those systems are compromised and we somehow someway get sick or have a physical ailment (like a sinus headache or an upset stomach or a cold), we often have been conditioned to immediately reach for over-the-counter medicine to "fix" the issue. The problem with this is we're loading our bodies with more toxins and synthetic agents that our bodies now have to spend valuable time and energy figuring out what to do with and filtering out of our system - wouldn't you rather have your body spend that time and energy healing itself? The truth is, Western medicine is amazing for trauma care, but it's not great for preventative or acute conditions - it often just masks the symptoms without addressing the underlying cause. What most people don't realize is that medication, whether prescription or over-the-counter, is created in a lab to mimic what was originally found in nature. That's right, medication aims to mimic the natural chemical constituents of plants. When we realize this, we can ask ourselves why not just go right to nature instead and avoid all the potential side effects? It does need to be mentioned that I'm talking about acute conditions - the occasional stomach upset, head tension, etc. For bigger health issues and if you're on prescription medication, I would absolutely recommend seeing your doctor or seeking out a functional medicine doctor (if you're looking for a great one, check out my functional medicine ninja doctor in the Expert Interview following this chapter - she can help you even if you aren't local to her office.) For clarity's sake, I'm not telling you to stop taking any kind of medication in lieu of an Eastern medicine modality unless you're working with some kind of medical professional to do so. Sidenote - another integrative medical option (integrative being a blend of Eastern and Western medicine practices) is to seek out a Prime Meridian Healthcare clinic, if there's one in your area. You can go to www.pmhclinic.com for more information.

<u>How?</u>

Some people choose to use herbs, some people choose food, some choose to use essential oils, others choose tinctures, while some people choose all of the above. Personally, I've always preferred to use essential oils just because they're so easy and convenient. With oils, they're simple to use and you can keep them right on/in your desk, purse, bag, etc. What I've found most often in the work settings are common disturbances like an upset stomach, headache, lack of energy, lack of focus and stress. While it's always important to know what caused these things, having a tool to help you in the moment so it doesn't ruin your whole day is crucial too. Just like anything else, you'll want to be your own best advocate on the oils you choose to use, so make sure to do your research - if you don't know where the plants were grown, what kind of testing and transparency the company has, if the testing isn't available for you to view, etc. don't spend your hard earned money on it. If you'd like some guidance here, take a peek at the Resources section - I have a free guide I'd be happy to send you. As a general rule though, while there are many different oils that can help with many different things, some of my favorites are using peppermint to help relieve head tension and upset stomachs, while it can also give you an energy boost and help with focus. I rub a drop or two on topically, diluting the essential oil with a carrier oil, and/or inhaling the aroma from my hands - if these are foreign terms to you, make sure you get the guide I mentioned before, I go through these things. For stress, I love smelling citrus oils - they're like natural sunshine in a bottle! I also love oils because there are so many scientifically researched books available to help you use them (though most leave the 26 letter science-y words out and use layman's terms instead!)

<u>Personal development books/audio/podcasts</u>

<u>Why?</u>

Self-care and self-growth always starts with us. I saw one of those Instagram photos someone shared once that said "Self-love is not only what you eat. It's what you watch, what you listen to, what you read, the people you hang around. Be mindful of all the things you put into your body emotionally, spiritually and physically." This is why this matters so much. Sometimes we can't always physically surround ourselves with people who inspire us, but we absolutely can choose what we put our time, attention and focus on/into by choosing wisely what we read, watch and listen to.

<u>How?</u>

What area of your life are you really interested in? Your health? Bettering your marriage? Creating a more positive mindset? Check out the Resources section in the back of the book for some of my favorite books that might just rock your world the way it did mine. Once you know what area of your life you'd like to focus on, do a little research and see what podcasts or books grab your attention.

<u>**Tongue Scraping**</u>

<u>Why?</u>

Most people are familiar with the backside of the toothbrush that usually has some kind of tongue brusher on it. The intention is there, but the result, not really so much. You're kind of just moving the particles on your tongue around, not really totally getting it all off. The idea of tongue scraping comes from Ayurveda, India's ancient medical system. During the course of the day and while we sleep, our tongues get coated with "ama," toxins basically. All things hygiene aside - which by the way, is a really great reason to tongue scrape all on its own - our mouths are the gateways to the rest of our bodies. Ever hear of oral health being directly linked to heart health? Tongue scraping is a way to get all that toxic crud off your tongue every day. Tongue scraping is also very beneficial for your digestion. When we eat, our taste buds send a signal to our digestive system to tell it what we just ate so it can release the proper digestive enzymes to break the food down (pretty cool huh?!), but when our tongues have a toxic coating, your taste buds can't always do their job. What do you say we give our bodies a hand here?

<u>How?</u>

A tongue scraper looks like a long, thin piece of stainless steel bent in a U shape with handles on either end. The idea is to use the scraper to pull off the coating on your tongue. Remember that the idea isn't to dig down into your tongue and pull off skin or damage anything in your mouth, but just with a little light pressure putting the scraper around the top of your tongue and pulling it down and out of your mouth from back to front. I usually do this over the sink. There are lots of variations on when to tongue scrape - some people do it before brushing, some do it after, while some do it first thing in the morning before they do anything else. Ayurveda is a really cool world to look into, with lots of good resources if you're interested. A lot of our "newer" practices like oil pulling are actually from Ayurveda, so it's actually not a new concept at all. It's just becoming more mainstream because people are starting to see how much great stuff we really can incorporate into our lives. If you're still a little fuzzy on how to tongue scrape, do a Google search and watch a video.

Herbal Tea

Why?

Herbal tea is incredibly soothing to your body, especially your nervous system. Choosing tea for people can be a little tough because there are so many different varieties. If the tea world is something that interests you, I would absolutely invite you to pick up a book on herbalism. The world of herbs can be mind-blowing! There's something comforting and calming about a hot cup of tea in your hands after a long day that just settles your mind and soothes your soul. Tea and a good book, anyone?

How?

Again, this is something I'm going to tell you to allow your body to choose. What do you need right now? If you want something that will help relax you, reach for some organic chamomile or lavender tea. If you're looking for something more refreshing, try a hibiscus or mint tea. You can buy loose tea to put in a strainer (great option if you get into creating your own tea concoctions), or you can buy tea in filter bags. As with everything you put on or in your body, I'm always going to suggest you buy organic. I know it's more expensive, but it makes a difference in your health. A huge difference. Your body doesn't need more toxins to filter out, our normal daily life is full of them as it is.

Dr. Brianne Holmes, Owner of Integrative Brain and Body

<u>About:</u>

Dr. Brianne Holmes is a chiropractor who practices Functional Medicine at Integrative Brain and Body. Integrative Brain and Body specializes in providing patients with answers to chronic health conditions with specialized lab work and lifestyle changes. She can be reached at her practice at 630-968-7891 or via email admin@ibrainandbody.com.

<u>Interview:</u>

What ramifications for a lack of self-care do you see most often in workplace settings?

1. The biggest ramification we see is what people are now terming "burnout." Energy is at an all-time low, you're exhausted all the time and exhaustion leads to other poor health choices. Extra caffeine or stimulants, staying up too late to get more work done due to lack of focus during the day, sacrificing sleep, sacrificing exercise and now due to fatigue and time constraints you are left to quick easy food choices that lack nutrients and will ultimately make the burn out worse.

What method of self-care do you personally feel is most important and/or effective for the general population, especially as it pertains to something they can do in the workplace setting?

It's hard to pick just one important method of self-care as there are so many small things a person can do that are all extremely important. So instead of picking just one method I'd like to apply a metaphor if that's OK: "put on your own oxygen mask first." We often put our own needs aside thinking that this type of dedication will eventually "pay off." Sure, you may get a raise or get rewarded, but the sacrifices you made will eventually add up and stop you from being able to move forward within the business. My practice is FULL of patients who have put the business ahead of their own health. This has led to gastrointestinal issues, adrenal issues, thyroid problems, skin diseases, autoimmune conditions, headaches/migraines, and feeling betrayed by your own body because it's falling apart.

In your ideal world, what would workplace wellness look like in every company?

Workplace wellness would look like a support system where the company leaders recognize and value their employee's health. I've seen companies who encourage their employees to participate in health challenges and reward them with paid days off, bonuses, gift cards and so on. If an employee is trying to get ahead in a company, or is competing with other employees for a better position, they aren't going to opt for these healthy changes just because someone like myself is giving them the warning of burn out. We live in a world of "this will never happen to me." The concern for their health has to come from higher up with an added reward system. Since we are all a bit shortsighted when it comes to our own health, the reward system is absolutely necessary. It gives the employee the instant gratification that we all crave. This in the long run will prevent "burn out" and create a stable work environment with healthy employees.

Chapter 3 - Ponderments

Notes, ah-ha's, braindumps, moments of clarity, interesting ideas:

What are some easy ways to be more in tune with your body's needs?

Is there anything you can foresee that might get in the way of this? What can you do to avoid that potential roadblock?

Chapter 4 - Rest as Medicine

We know how important sleep is, yet with all the responsibilities on our shoulders, we're lucky if we get a fraction of the good, quality sleep we need each night. Now obviously I'm not talking about those secret naps you take on your lunch break or at your desk (wink wink), but I'm talking about the sleep you get every night. The truth is, how your day flows is directly related to not only how well you slept the night before, but how your evening flowed into your sleep cycle. I'll break this down for you so you can get some different ideas on how to set yourself up for a great day the night before. So really, let's answer this question - how can I rest better at night? The idea with these suggestions is to create a bit of a self-care routine that literally signals to your brain "it's time to start getting ready for bed!"

Set a schedule and know how many hours you need

Why?

Our bodies really dig routines. If you're already doing this, you'll agree. I've gotten my body into the habit of going to bed around 9:30pm and being up around 6:15am (my body loves 8-9 hours of sleep, and I try to give it that whenever possible). What ends up happening is you start to have a natural alarm clock.

Has this ever happened to you? Your body gets in a rhythm and a lot of the time, as if by magic, your body wakes up minutes before your alarm goes off and at night, your body naturally gets really sleepy around the time you're accustomed to going to sleep.

<u>How?</u>

Getting your body into this rhythm can be a little tricky and it takes some trial and error. My suggestion is to pay attention to the number of hours you sleep and know when you feel the best and most rested. I've met people who swear they only need 6 hours and others who feel like zombies unless they've had 7 or 8. Know that the quality of sleep, not just the quantity, you get also plays a huge factor in how you feel, so take note of that as well. If you feel like you need 9 hours, but that's because you wake up wide awake for an hour in the middle of the night, that's something to consider. Luckily, this whole section is geared towards finding ways to help your body sleep better during the night. Once you know how many hours of sleep your body requires, you now know what time you need to go to bed to wake up on time, get ready for work without haste, etc. Once you know what time you need to go to bed, it's now on you to give your body that whenever possible. Don't hate me, but I'm going to invite you to keep the same sleep schedule on your off days too - reason being is if you try to mess with your schedule on a weekend, it's going to take you a few days once the work week hits to get you back into your normal pattern, just to slam into another weekend. The idea here is to help your body get on a sleep schedule that you try to keep at all costs. Obviously, certain things can't be helped, and you may not always be able to be in bed at your normal time, but try to make those occasions as rare as possible, if you can.

Prep for the next day the night before

Why?

We'll cover more of this in the next chapter, but making a conscious effort to prep things for the next day (coffee maker, your clothes, your lunch, etc.) can make your morning go so much smoother and prevent last-minute rushing around.

How?

Know what you need for the next day and get it ready the evening before. For example, if you bring your lunch to work each day, make it and pack it the night before so you can just grab it from the fridge on your way out. If you spend quite a bit of time in your closet in the morning trying to figure out what to wear, choose it the evening before and have it ready to go for the morning. See where I'm going with this? A little effort in preparation can save you tons of time and energy in frustration and hurrying the next morning.

Baths

<u>Why?</u>

Taking a hot bath at night is an amazing way to unwind, take some time for yourself, soak away stress and just relax for a little while. This can be an amazing way to prepare your body for sleep as well, since it's a nice and relaxing way to transition from your day into sleeping.

<u>How?</u>

If you don't have a bathtub, I'm going to give you an idea that I have to trust you're not going to laugh at. Hey, desperate times call for desperate measures! If you find yourself sans a bathtub (like if you only have a stand-up shower to work with), plug the drain in your sink and fill it with water at the temperature you'd like. You're going to create a mini-bath to soak your feet in. Yes, I'm telling you to sit on your bathroom counter and stick your feet into the sink. Get crazy and put your hands in there too. Regardless what you're working with, you can create this bath as sort of a ritual - it can look the same each time, or it can look completely different. Some people love to add Epsom salts in their baths to help soothe achy muscles. Some people find luxury in bubbles. Some love to put essential oils based on their needs for the day into their bath water (like lavender or a tree oil like frankincense). Some love to put a few drops of a carrier oil in their water, like fractionated coconut oil or avocado oil, so their skin is getting some additional nourishment. Others like to add flower petals and light candles, while some like to do it all! Whatever your definition of luxury and relaxation looks like, make this experience all about you. Focus on your breathing by taking some deep breaths to settle in and help your mind become still.

Evening Routine

Why?

I love the idea of having end-caps to your day - a way to start the day and a way to end the day, every day. An evening routine just means you have certain things you're doing for yourself each night before you close your eyes to sleep. It could be the same routine every night, it could be different each night. The idea is that you're giving yourself a certain amount of time to really nourish YOU and prep your body for a good night's rest.

How?

To me, there are two things that are important when deciding how to do this. One is deciding how much time you'd like to have and the other is deciding what you'd like to do during that time (or deciding NOT to have a plan and allow your body to choose what it wants/needs each night). It could be 15 minutes, or it could be an hour. Everyone's life is different and has different circumstances, so do what works for you. Some ideas of what your evening routine could include could be daily hygienic things like taking a shower or a bath, brushing your teeth, washing your face, etc. It could include giving yourself a relaxing self-massage with coconut oil and your favorite relaxing essential oil. It could be reading, meditating, connecting with your spouse or significant other, working on your breathing. What it shouldn't include though is anything with a screen. One of the worst things you can do before you go to sleep is look at a screen - so disconnect from the TV, computer screen, smart watch and smartphone at least an hour or two before bedtime. There are a couple different reasons for this - one is the light from the screen signaling to your brain that it's daytime and that you should be awake. This can make your systems think they need to be "on" instead of winding down for sleep. The second is the influx of information being received from these devices. We've all been there - we're just getting ready to go to bed, we're so sleepy, we check our phones one last time and see that email or text message and all of a sudden, our brain is now going a million miles an hour. Make your evening time

YOUR time, for you, without the world's tragedies of the day, without scrolling through everyone's fantastic lives according to social media. Just you. The name of the game here is setting boundaries.

Get your inner caveman/cavewoman on

Why?

The idea of your bedroom should be that of a cave. Cool and dark. The ideal temperature to sleep at for most people is usually 67 degrees, as our body temperature rises when we're sleeping and I'm sure we've all woken up at some point dripping in sweat and not being able to go back to sleep from the heat. Not fun. Keeping your bedroom completely dark though, that might be a new concept. The idea is to not allow any outside influences to disrupt your sleep. Lights, electromagnetic waves from TV's, phones, etc. can all be huge sleep disturbances.

How?

If it lights up, it gets turned off or it gets kicked out of the room all together. I'm talking TV's, phones, lights, all of it. If the idea of taking the TV out of your room swore you off of me all together, I get it - I know the TV can be a deal-breaker for some. What I'd invite you to do is start with everything else. If you have an attached bathroom, leave your phone charging in your bathroom. Use the alarm clock on your phone in there instead of the old ones that light up (ever wake up in the middle of the night and stare at the time on your alarm clock for hours? Yeah, not helpful). If there are street lights or any kind of light that shines in your windows, maybe get some blackout curtains to keep the light out. The idea here is to make your room as dark as possible to set your body up for a restful night's sleep and minimize any chances of disturbances.

Keep a journal or notebook by your bedside

Why?

If you're like me, sometimes your head hits the pillow and gets flooded with things you forgot to do, thoughts, emotions, or sometimes you have a dream and when you wake up from it you think, "I'll totally remember that tomorrow!" only to wake up and forget the whole thing even happened (especially disappointing when you have dreams about loved ones who have passed on).

How?

Anytime anything flows into your mind, write it down in your journal/notebook so you can refer back to it the next day. Sometimes hanging onto those thoughts in an effort not to forget can cause you to not sleep so well. What a lot of people have found benefit in as well is doing what I call a "braindump" before bed and this is literally just taking a journal, notebook or piece of paper and doing free-writing of all the thoughts, feelings, to-do's, accomplishments, failures, all the things that happened that day, just to literally dump it out of your brain so it doesn't keep you awake at night. Now let's be honest, I'm not telling you that dumping it out on paper is going to make whatever it is go away or feel any better, but there's this energetic release that happens when you literally spill out thoughts you're holding onto in your brain by handwriting it on paper. Try it out, it's cathartic if nothing else. PS - if you don't like the thought of writing things down for fear of people finding it, consider writing it all down and then ripping up the paper into tiny pieces and throwing it away or burying the tiny shreds in the Earth weekly, or placing it in the shredder. The act of tearing, shredding, burying or burning it can actually be a great form of release - like you're giving it all away to a higher power, the good and the bad.

Morning Routine

Why?

Just like the evening routine, the morning routine is something you do every morning to start your day off. In contrast to the evening routine where the idea is to incorporate things into your routine to wind down, the intention of the morning routine is to help energize and start your day off on the right foot and also to help ground or balance you for the day ahead. Over the years I've found it much easier to be consistent with a morning routine than an evening routine. No one does anything perfectly, we're all a work in progress.

<u>How?</u>

What starts your morning off right? What sets you up for the best day ever? How does it feel when you do something that totally connects you to yourself? Just like the evening routine, decide how much time you want to give yourself for your morning routine. This time is just for you to really fill your cup for the day. Maybe it's 15 minutes, maybe it's an hour, maybe it's 2 hours. It's unique to you! What do you want this time to be filled with? Some ideas could be just sitting in silence, drinking tea or coffee and really just focusing on all the good things that have already happened in your day (like you woke up breathing), if you're religious, you could read from your religious text, you could meditate or do some breathing exercises. You could also do some physical exercises or yoga, stretching, journaling, drinking water - any and all of these ideas are amazing, but know this is only the tip of the iceberg. Do what fills your cup up and keep doing it every single day. I love making sure a morning routine is something I can take with me anywhere I am, like if

I'm traveling. You'll be surprised how much your day is affected when you DON'T get to do your morning routine. I know when I'm in a space where I can't do mine or can't do it as intently or effectively as I want (like if I'm traveling and staying with a group), I feel all kinds of wonky and off for the whole day.

<u>Expert Interview</u>

Nicole Martin, Owner of HRBoost

<u>About:</u>

Nicole Martin is an internationally renowned speaker, author, and CEO and Founder of HRBoost, LLC. Nicole is a dynamic and empowering consultative leader and futurist skilled in helping organizations meet their strategic objectives through their people. As a highly regarded and sought-after expert, her knowledge and advice have been featured in newspapers and magazines throughout the country. Recent publications in which she has been seen include Forbes.com, the Daily Herald Business Ledger, and Fast Company. She is the author of the books The Talent Emergency, The Human side of Profitability and The Power of Joy and Purpose.

In addition, Nicole is the host of the internet TV show HR in the Fast Lane.

<u>Interview:</u>

What ramifications for a lack of self-care do you see most often in workplace settings?

A lack of self-care can lead to a number of impacts in the workplace and the most common is surely job burnout. Talent can be overly taxed in a tight labor market and a lack of intentional balance between work and personal demands can lead to stressors that can negate self-care from the equation. Anyone who takes on a heavy workload to include overtime hours is at risk. Some try to be everything to everyone and people who work in supportive roles, like healthcare for example, are at higher risk. Nonetheless, everyone is vulnerable to job burnout when self-care is neglected. And honestly, this is the least of the consequences. Ironically, most do not take a proactive approach to self-care when they are fast tracking in business and career development.

What method of self-care do you personally feel is most important and/or effective for the general population, especially as it pertains to something they can do in the workplace setting?

The workplace can be where most people spend a great deal of time. Traditional work environments set forth a number of standard dynamics in recent decades that can leave people feeling powerless. When people have been managed as though they have little influence on their job it can cascade into dysfunction it their lives. This must change. For example, when an adult can do little to control their schedule, their assignments, the pace of their workload or access resources to be effective, how can we expect them to feel empowered on any level. The reality is that workplaces can help to prevent the feeling of powerlessness at work. Strategies like job enrichment, well-being while at work and accountable culture management are opportunities to create work environments where people actually enjoy coming to work. Ensuring managers are developed to be managers of choice could mean that organizational leadership has a chance to be modeled in the workplace. Managers of Choice are developed with emotional intelligence and skill for relationship building, trust building, skill building, organization brand building and bottom line, they care. Any organization that does not proactively invite talent to make a collaborative contribution all the while providing resources and empowerment strategies to allow talent to excel on all levels is missing a valuable advantage to capture innovation and productivity in the workplace.

In your ideal world, what would workplace wellness look like in every company?

Brene Brown's research findings for how to live a wholehearted life, showed that "things … like rest and play, are as vital to our health as nutrition and exercise." Yet how often do people treat this as their personal responsibility to deliver this in their life?

With over 50% of the talent pool moving into a freelance workforce by 2027, it seems many have taken self-care into their own hands. Talent seeks to be empowered to be trusted to do their work regardless of where it gets done. At the same time, people are the first to neglect their own health.

Ideally, every person should have the education of nutrition. Ideally, every person should have a coach, someone that cared to check in and ask how often they rest and play, how often they feel invigorated. Any organization that takes time to care about a person on a whole level is taking a step in the right direction. The beginning of this paradigm shift in the workplace has begun, but still only 9% implement proactive wellness initiatives globally. The first fundamental shift is to create an environment of choice and empowerment. When people are empowered, informed and then able to choose, only then can self-care take hold in the workplace. And why is all of this important? Because we need people and people need to be well in order to do their jobs well. And everyone, deserves joy and purpose through work.

Chapter 4 - Ponderments

Notes, ah-ha's, braindumps, moments of clarity, interesting ideas:

What can you do, starting tonight to help yourself truly rest better?

____

____

____

____

____

____

____

____

____

____

____

____

____

____

____

Is there anything you can foresee that might get in the
way of this? What can you do to avoid that potential
roadblock?

Chapter 5 - Preparation for Sanity

Like I mentioned in the last chapter when we briefly talked about prepping for the next day the night before, a little effort spent prepping for your day and/or your week could pay dividends in time and energy day to day. One of the best kept secrets I had when I worked in an office was spending some time on Sundays prepping things for the whole week - it just made my week flow so much smoother and made me feel like I wasn't rushing to get things done each day.

An idea if "prepping" or "routine" isn't really your thing - get comfortable using your digital calendar and/or note-taking app. When a thought comes into your head like "we're out of apples!" you can set a reminder to put it on your shopping list (if you don't use a digital shopping list already). These are great options for those random thoughts that pop into our heads which we don't want to lose - dump them into your note taking app or set a reminder to do the thing you forgot you needed to do.

The question you must be asking yourself is "so what are some things I can prep ahead of time to make my work week flow better?" I'm going to keep this section a little shorter since most of these are self-explanatory.

A note about these ideas - you can absolutely do these things the night before, but sometimes it's even more of a benefit to do them the day or evening before your work week even starts. For example, if you're someone who takes supplements and/or medication in the morning or evening, instead of just prepping this the evening before, you could prep them for the whole week - that way all you have to do is just remember to take them each day!

<u>Prep anything that will help you feel calm each day</u>

- Lunch

- Dinner

- Clothes

- Your schedule for the week (kid's practices, doctor's appointments, dates, dinners out, etc.)

- Coffee/Tea maker

- Supplements/medication

- Make sure your vehicle has gas

<u>Expert Interview</u>

<u>ComPsych, provider of employee assistance and wellness programs</u>

<u>About:</u>

ComPsych Corporation is the world's largest provider of employee assistance programs (EAP) and is the pioneer and worldwide leader of fully integrated EAP, behavioral health, wellness, work-life, HR, FMLA and absence management services under its GuidanceResources® brand. ComPsych provides services to more than 50,000 organizations covering more than 109 million individuals throughout the U.S. and 160 countries. By creating "build-to-suit" programs, ComPsych helps employers attract and retain employees, increase employee productivity and improve overall health and well-being. For more information, please visit www.compsych.com

<u>Interview:</u>

What ramifications for a lack of self-care do you see most often in workplace settings?

The most common consequences for lack of self-care are strained relationships at work, heightened stress levels, less energy, difficulty concentrating and making decisions and ultimately, job burnout.

What method of self-care do you personally feel is most important and/or effective for the general population, especially as it pertains to something they can do in the workplace setting?

The most promising mode of self-care is mindfulness training. This can be used to manage stress, promote a positive outlook, inspire better relationships with colleagues and increase focus and productivity at work. ComPsych teaches employees to stay present, worry less (be "less affected and more effective") and multi-task less, which can increase both enjoyment and performance at work.

In your ideal world, what would workplace wellness look like in every company?

The ideal workplace wellness initiative would include the elements of physical, mental, financial and even social wellness. By supporting the whole person, wellness can address life challenges, promote personal growth and help employees be more engaged at work and throughout life in general.

Chapter 5 - Ponderments

Notes, ah-ha's, braindumps, moments of clarity, interesting ideas:

What are some ideas of things you could do to help you feel more prepared and allow your week to flow smoothly?

____

____

____

____

____

____

____

____

____

____

____

____

____

____

____

____

____

Is there anything you can foresee that might get in the
way of this? What can you do to avoid that potential
roadblock?

____

____

____

____

____

____

____

____

____

____

____

____

____

____

____

____

____

____

Chapter 6 - Zen Your Space for Calm Clarity

Let's face it, you're going to be sitting in the same office/cubicle/desk day in and day out for (hopefully) a long time to come. You might as well spruce up the joint to fill it with positive vibes and feel like a place you actually want to be in! While I'm going to give you some suggestions, you'll want to make sure the things you want to do are ok by your company's policies - some places are more lenient than others.

So, the question you might be asking yourself is "How do I create a space of calm in a cubicle/office/desk when I might possibly have restrictions in freedom on what to do?" So glad you asked! Also, just a side note - the idea of "Zen your space" could easily apply to another space in your life, like your vehicle for example. How can you make a space you spend a lot of time in have better energy and make you feel happier spending time in it? This is especially important for those commuters or field workers who spend a lot of time in their vehicles. Phoebe, my love-scuffed 2008 Toyota 4Runner, and I have had many-a days, meals, adventures (both planned and frighteningly unplanned), laughs, tears and conversations together - she's family :).

<u>Change your computer screensaver and/or background</u>

<u>Why?</u>

Because how fun is it to wake your computer up and see one of your favorite photos or scenes staring back at you?! I know plenty of people who love walking by other people's computers just so they can see their screensaver or background because it just makes them happy. Who knew your memory or your dream could make someone else excited, nostalgic or happy too?!

<u>How?</u>

You can do this any way you want. You can choose a photo of a family member, significant other or spouse, pet, a memory from your favorite vacation, etc. OR you can choose something that will be happening in the future - like if you're getting married, going on vacation or getting a new vehicle you can choose a photo that will make you excited for that upcoming thing!

<u>Include plants or flowers on your desk or in your space</u>

<u>Why?</u>

It's a known fact that plants give us oxygen, so they help clean the air essentially. They can smell amazing, bring in some grounding vibes because they're of the

Earth and remind us that amazing things can grow from a single seed.

How?

The plants or flowers you choose can be symbolic – if you want to feel surrounded in love, you could choose freshcut flowers in a vase each week, or you bring a potted flower to put on your desk. Same thing with other plants, this is completely of your choosing, if your company allows it.

Keep something fun and childlike in/on your desk

How?

When I worked in an office, I kept a little tub of Playdoh on my desk. It reminded me of my childhood and every time I looked at it or took it out, the smell and the squishiness took me back to simpler times. That's the idea here - connecting to your inner child.

How?

What did you love to play with when you were younger? Legos? Playdoh? Is there a way you can bring a little piece of that back to your adult life? Sometimes just holding something in your hand like a touchstone can be so cathartic to the soul during stressful times. Even just the sight of something can elicit the same emotions.

<u>**Create a vision board**</u>

<u>Why?</u>

While vision boards have become more and more popular, it can still be a foreign term for a lot of people. A vision board is basically a collection of photos and/or words (or anything else really) that help you visualize your ideal life. Your goals, your dreams - who you want to be, what you want to do and have. Sometimes on life's hard days, your vision board can be an inspirational reminder of why you're doing what you're doing and motivate you to keep going.

<u>How?</u>

You can go at creating a vision board yourself of course, a lot of people grab a bunch of magazines and start ripping out images or words that align with their ideal life they want to create. Vacations they want to take, goals they have, it all gets put on the visionboard. If you're interested, I lead a more in-depth online vision boarding workshop that you can access. Details on this workshop are in the Resources section of this book, I'd love to have you in there!

<u>Diffuser for aromatherapy</u>

<u>Why?</u>

In lieu of candles or other scented things, I'm going to invite you to opt for an essential oil diffuser with some essential oils. Candles aren't usually allowed in offices due to fire hazards, and the same thing goes for things you plug in - sometimes all scents aren't welcome in office settings due to sensitivities. You'll have to know your own atmosphere here. The other thing with candles and other options with scents (plug-ins, tart warmers, etc.) is whatever is inside is almost always synthetic and therefore toxic to our systems. If your company would allow you an essential oil diffuser, you can diffuse pure plant essential oils (that is, the essential oil that is taken right from the plant and bottled without adding anything else). These diffusers can be water based that plug in (if allowed), there are also car diffusers and USB diffuser options as well.

<u>How?</u>

Decide on the mood for the day. Is there a lot of stress and anxiousness in the air? Maybe diffuse something grounding, like a conifer tree oil such as Siberian Fir. Are you feeling a little sad or down? Maybe a citrus oil like wild orange can help boost your spirits. Are you feeling scattered and in need of some help focusing? Diffusing some lemon or peppermint essential oil is sure to help. I always invite people to use oils based on need, but don't discount diffusing an oil just because it smells amazing - that's a totally valid reason! If you're a little hazy on essential oils or aren't quite sure what to buy or how to use them, make sure you check out the Resources section in the back of this book for a gift from me to help you with just that.

Use Crystals/Stones

Why?

From healing-journeys-energy.com:

"Just like anything in nature, crystals and stones can be incredibly healing to be around - each with their own distinct uses and characteristics. The Earth's natural crystals have taken several hundreds of thousands to a few million years to form and grow and during this period of growth they have weathered the storms of Mother Earth's development, they've survived volcanic upheavals, the Ice Age as well as all the natural and man-made disasters thrown at them." Just like we've talked about getting our bodies out in nature, bringing nature INTO the office can also be another way to change the energy that surrounds you.

How?

Because there are so many different kinds of crystals and stones, it can be hard to choose. One option that I have grown to love most recently is rainbow fluorite. It's a beautiful stone to look at with its green, teal and purple interweaving, but rainbow fluorite is a natural stabilizer of energy. Keeping this stone in your pocket or on your desk can help you stabilize your own energy when you're in the midst of many people with many different types of energy. Some others I like to have around the office is clear quartz for focus, amethyst for stress relief and black tourmaline to keep negative energies away. There's so much more to the wonderful world of crystals, I truly invite you to dive more into the subject - maybe grab a couple books and see what speaks to you. Crystals and stones can be such an amazing tool in your self-care toolkit for physical and emotional concerns as well as spiritual healing!

Art

<u>Why?</u>

There's something so cathartic about creating something with your hands. This may or may not be something you'd be able to do at work, but it could be an extracurricular activity you could partake in. Creating something with your hands feels like being able to transmute the worries and stresses of the day into, well, some form of art. It's stress relief, it's creation, it's destruction, it's art without limits.

<u>How?</u>

What are you intensely interested in? Dancing? Drawing? Pottery? Jewelry making? Widdling? Mosaics? Photography? Writing? Whatever your preferred art form is, allow it to come back into your life in some way - maybe at an even greater capacity than it originally was. If you're up for it, take a new class or take a refresher class. If you don't know what your art is, how amazing is it that you get to go on the adventure of finding out? I love hopping on Groupon to look at the different class offerings nearby - you might be amazed at what you find that could spark a passion you didn't know existed! Another idea too - who do you know that's artsy? They might have an insider's scoop on where to go or they might even be open to teaching you themselves. The power of ask is always there for you.

<u>Expert Interview</u>

Laura Sage, Founder and CEO of Chill Chicago

<u>About:</u>

Chill's mission to help people live less stressed and more mindful lives (they hope you will join them in this pursuit). They have a beautiful studio that offers approachable modern mediation classes, no-need-to-get-naked massages and thoughtfully curated retail items. Want some Chill at your office? Chill Co has that covered. Want to take a deeper dive into mindfulness? Chill Ed offers certified meditation teacher training. Want to get away from it all? Chill Away is your source for mindful retreats. Come into Chill and leave less stressed.

For more information visit www.chillchicago.com.

Follow Chill on Instagram - @chill_out_chi / @hedgepink and on Facebook - Chill Meditation + Massage

<u>Interview:</u>

What ramifications for a lack of self-care do you see most often in workplace settings?

People don't take time to attend to their own mental health. We know how to eat properly and to exercise our bodies, but most people don't take time to exercise their brains, sleep enough or relax. Ramifications include burnout (which was recently classified as a disease by the World Health Organization), depression, anxiety and exhaustion.

What method of self-care do you personally feel is most important and/or effective for the general population, especially as it pertains to something they can do in the workplace setting?

Well, I'm biased towards meditation (in all its forms). What's great about meditation is that it's good for just about everyone. It's hard to find too many things, aside from oxygen and water, that you can say that about. And it's something people can do at home, while commuting and at work.

In your ideal world, what would workplace wellness look like in every company?

In an ideal world, workplace wellness would include both physical and mental wellness initiatives, and these initiatives would be customized based on each company's unique needs. Wellness is not one-size-fits-all.

Chapter 6 - Ponderments

Notes, ah-ha's, braindumps, moments of clarity, interesting ideas:

How can you bring more Zen and nature into your life at work?

____

____

____

____

____

____

____

____

____

____

____

____

____

____

____

Is there anything you can foresee that might get in the way of this? What can you do to avoid that potential roadblock?

Ever have those days when you need something to recalibrate you and QUICK?! I sometimes have those momentary bursts of anxiety, someone's words or energy throw me for a loop, times when I'm just not feeling my best and I just need something quick to align me again. Next time you're feeling a little off-kilter, test out one (or multiple) of these self-care tactics.

Smile at and/or give a pleasantry to a stranger

Look someone (or multiple people) in the eyes as you walk past each other, smile and say hello, good morning/afternoon/evening, have a nice day, etc.

Smiling, looking people in the eye and/or exchanging pleasantries with acquaintances or strangers can have an immediate boost in our mood (and you never know when your smile and kind gesture might actually change the course of someone else's day).

Gratitude - STAT

Take a time out and think of 5 things you're grateful for right now - not things that are going to happen, or "I'll be grateful when....," but real things right now - like your health, that your eyes can see, your lungs can breathe, you got to your office safely, you have a car to drive - go for the seemingly insignificant things, those are what most often can feel the best to be grateful for when you realize that you're among a minority in the world to have some of those things!

Breathe

Inhale for 5 counts, hold for 5 counts, exhale for 5 counts. Repeat as long as you need. This option is great for those instances of sparked anxiety when you need your mind and body to calm down.

Get fresh air outside in nature

Being in the same environment that triggered your need for a quick self-care tactic often won't help ease the flare up. If you're inside, get outside. If you're outside, go somewhere else that's outside. The idea here is you're going for fresh air and nature, just being present and breathing is key. This is my go-to when something happens and I'm near tears - I need to get out. Some might call it an escape, but I call it self-love and self-care.

Earthing

Going off of the last tip about getting outside, take your shoes off and put your feet in the grass while you're at it. If you don't want to take your shoes off or don't have time, put your hands on the grass, on a tree, in a natural body of water - something of the Earth. Imagine you're releasing and feeding whatever is happening to the Earth and asking it to fill you with light and loving energy, transmuting any negative or toxic thoughts, emotions and feelings into thoughts, emotions and feelings of love, peace, insert your own desires here.

Surprise Yourself

Don't think about the page, or the section, just open this book and whatever is on that page, choose from there. You can even close your eyes, open the book, point somewhere on one of the open pages and do that thing if you can.

Chapter 7 - Ponderments

Notes, ah-ha's, braindumps, moments of clarity, interesting ideas:

What is going to be your go-to self-care practice you'll use in a pinch?

Is there anything you can foresee that might get in the way of this? What can you do to avoid that potential roadblock?

Help! I'm Overwhelmed with Options!!

If you're new to self-care, all the ideas in this book can be a little, well, overwhelming. If you'd like my advice, my golden nuggets, the things I would absolutely recommend pulling from this book, here they are.... Drumroll please...

Morning Routine

Evening Routine

1 go-to technique from the book to de-stress your mind and body - just choose 1. Try it on for size, see how it fits. If you like it, keep it. If you don't, choose another one.

Rinse and repeat until you find what fits!

Resources the Author Recommends

Throughout the book I mentioned different people and tools letting you know I'd list additional info in the Resources section. These are modalities that I've personally used or created from my own experiences along my own self-care journey. I invite you to take a peek into each to see if they align with you and what you need.

Self-Care in the Workplace and Virtual Self-Care Workshops

Visit my website at www.loveyourlifewithmisty.com for to see all current offerings available for businesses of all sizes as well as workshops for individuals.

Essential Oils

Visit the Nature's Apothecary section of my website www.loveyourlifewithmisty.com/essentialoils for free videos, ebooks and other information.

Buy The Self-Care Survival Guide for Employees in bulk

The book you're holding makes for a wonderful gift for family, friends, coworkers and employees! Receive $5 off retail price when you buy in bulk, visit www. loveyourlifewithmisty.com/books to learn more.

<u>Connect with me on social media for more self-care tips</u>

Facebook /Instagram - loveyourlifewithmisty

LinkedIn - Love Your Life with Misty

<u>Favorite personal development books</u>

These are books I turn to time and time again when I'm in need of personal growth and development in different areas of my life. Read the descriptions of each, see what resonates. Usually, I find that if a book has me all "yessssssss!!!!" within the first 10 pages or so, it's something I need at that point in my life. I've often picked up books that I just couldn't get into at the time only to pick them back up a year or more later and they totally rock my world. Go with what speaks to you in the season of life that you're in.

It's Not Your Money by Tosha Silver

Firestarter Sessions by Danielle LaPorte

Warrior Goddess Training by HeatherAsh Amara

Artist's Way by Julia Cameron

The Game of Life and How to Play It by Florence Scovel Shinn

Reveal by Meggan Watterson

Ending Gratitude

Regardless the role you have played in my life - be it family, friend, romantic partner, energy healer, business connection, acquaintance, reader, workshop attendee or someone who sent me a message once 5 years ago on social media - you have somehow someway contributed your energy to the creation of this book.

While I can't start naming names because I'll inevitably forget someone, I do need to specifically thank my parents - biological and not. Alive and on the other side. It's because of you I've never given up on what my heart told me to do, even when I chose all the long roads. Even when I fell flat on my face each time. You're the brightest lights in my life and I'm so grateful to have you. I love you all so very much. Thank you for always being examples to me and allowing me to be a conglomerate of you all.

This was a collection of desires people have been asking for and I'm so grateful and honored to have somehow been guided to be the conduit to bring it to life. The love and excitement I've felt from you for this book has filled every crevice of my being, from more places and people than I ever could have imagined.

Even if you and I have never met or connected in any way, your desire for a resource like this was felt so strongly that a seed was planted for its creation.

For all of this, for all of you, I am forever grateful. Thank you. Truly.

I'll leave you with a small, but powerful prayer that has helped me tremendously through the years while learning the hard lessons of caring for myself and releasing what no longer serves me to create space for even better things to come into my life.

My desire is for it to find whomever might need it.

From the author, Tosha Silver:

Let everything that needs to go, let it go,

Let everything that needs to stay, let it stay.

Let everything that needs to come, let it come.

Wishing you the most magical process of falling in love with yourself, your life and the world around you.

Sending you so much love!

Misty

Dedication

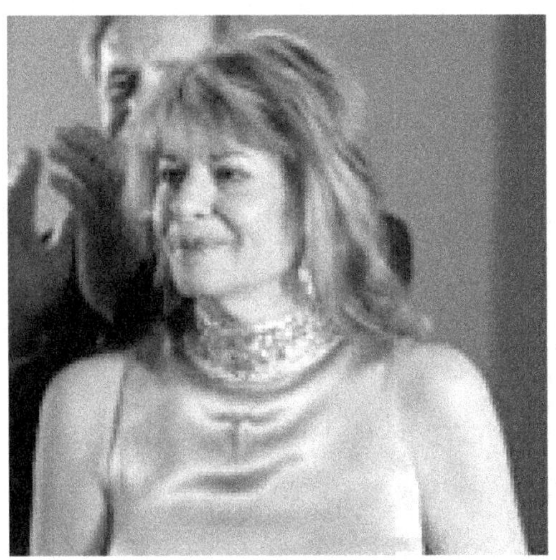

The creation of this book is in honor of my beautiful angel mama, Cathy Hudek, and the legacy she left for all of us.

About a year after my mom passed, I went to see a friend. I'll never forget something my friend told me. She said when you lose your mother, it is often the most intensely soul-crushing pain of your life because you have lost the anchor that held you in this world. You've lost the person who quite literally brought you into this life and without them physically in this world, you can feel like you've lost your place.

My mom's story is very long and very deep, but suffice it to say this woman was and is my greatest teacher in life, and as it pertains to this book - in health. Through her struggles and illness, surgeries and lifestyle choices, she gave me the gift of a front row seat to the visual representation of how precious our health is and what a gift it is that we get the choice to care for ourselves each and every day. Without her inspiration and guidance from the other side, this book most surely may never have been birthed.

Mark Batterson wrote in his book, *Chase the Lion*, "Your greatest legacy isn't your dream. Your greatest legacy is the next generation of dreamers that your dream inspires - the dream within a dream. Our dreams predate us. They were born long before we were. Our dreams postdate us. They make a difference long after we are gone." My mother was the wildest dreamer you'd ever meet and I'm so grateful all of her dreams, wild ideas and adventures... her legacy... can live on through me.

Helping others connect with themselves and the world around them is a special kind of catharsis for my own soul. As you heal, I heal, as I heal, you heal, as we heal, she heals - and that's how the world heals. One by one, but as a collective.